Who Cares

A Loving Guide for Caregivers

*Providing future caregivers the most
important facts about my life*

Dee Marrella

PRESS

A Division of the Diogenes Consortium

SANFORD • FLORIDA

This guide is intended as a means for the user to create a journal of their life's events and to share personal thoughts with its readers. before taking any action that could have legal ramifications, discuss such matters with an attorney of your choice. Likewise, before taking any action effecting your health care, discuss those actions with your personal physician.

Published by DC Press
2445 River Tree Circle
Sanford, FL 32771
http://www.focusonethics.com

This book was set in Adobe Novarese
Cover Design and Composition by Jonathan Pennell

Library of Congress Catalog Number: Applied for
          Marrella. Dee,
Who Cares
          ISBN: 0-9708444-8-4

First DC Press Edition
10   9   8   7   6   5   4   3
Printed in the United States of America

This book is lovingly dedicated
to my mother, Beatrice Delia —
A happy person who suffered so much
in her later years.

To my sisters,
Terry Nicoletti and Karen Wiesen —
Together, we tried our very best.

To my daughters, Tammy Toso,
Lani Martin and Robin Russo —
Your love and support during a very
trying time will never be forgotten.

To the love of my life, Len —
You encouraged me to care for my
Mom. You shared my stress and pain.
For this I am forever grateful.

To the older generation —
You taught me so many of life's most
important lessons.

CONTENTS

v
— **Preface** —

xvii
— **Caveat** —

xix
— **Introduction** —

xxv
— **Publisher's Comment** —

1
— **Part I** —
General Instructions

A letter to my future caregivers

Major medical decisions

21

— Part II —
Priorities for Care Medical information

Nursing home/alternative care priorities

Providers of services

(medical, legal, hygienic, other)

List of those preferred

List of those to be avoided

49

— Part III —
My Preferences

Food likes and dislikes

Product likes and dislikes

Entertainment likes and dislikes

Clothing preferences and sizes

Personal hygiene and care

Special treats

Things I want to keep

83
— Part IV —
Who Am I?

My fears

My personality

113
— Part V —
Relationships

Friends

Visits

Gifts

Conversational topics

Places to go together

Special treats

119

— **Part VI** —
Holiday and Religious Observance

Secular holidays — observance and celebration

Family occasions — observance and celebration

Religious affiliation

Attendance, participation and frequency

Ritual and practice

Degree of importance, priorities

129

— **Part VII** —
Important Names

My generation

Previous generations

Children and grandchildren

Nieces and nephews

Friends

Associates

145

— **Part VIII** —
Financial and Business Affairs

169

— **Part IX** —
Life's Lessons

What I have learned in my life

and would like to pass along to

my loved ones

PREFACE

How I came to write this guide.

*F*OR A YEAR AND A HALF I had been visiting my 93-year-old mother in a nursing home. Never did I think I would have to face the heartbreak and guilt of seeing my Mom helpless and in a wheelchair. Nor was I prepared for the heartbreak I would feel for those around her.

Some sights will never leave me:

🌹 A woman sitting in the hallway, purse in hand, never moving from her particular chair, waiting for someone to come for her — all day, every day, for months.

A handsome man in his eighties — father of twelve children — eagerly waiting for the Christmas holidays, hoping to see any of his children. Not one showed up...not until his death a few weeks later. (Was his heart broken?)

A short, humped-back, older woman constantly walking the halls all alone — never talking to anyone, never visited. When she sat near other residents, she was chased away. As she walked passed, she was taunted. She just kept walking.

A lovely lady in her fifties who came to visit her mother — a victim of Alzheimer's. Sometimes she looked so tired, just coming from her own job. She had a brother, but he never visited his mother. He rationalized that his mother had actually died years earlier. (I wondered — if he suffered from the same disease — would his mother have come to visit him? I'm sure she would have gone every day possible to lovingly care for him.)

I could go on with such stories. There is heartbreak on both sides. Parents are getting older and more helpless. Children are trying to cope with the worry, exhaustion and guilt.

I loved my mother very much. My mother loved me very much. I know there are many of you who feel the same — you love your parents, you love your children. Sitting at the nursing home, observing all of these things, I saw how quickly the years can overtake us, how little time might be left before we become "the older generation" — the ones in need of caregivers.

If I have my wish, my children will not have to face the worry and heartache I felt as a caregiver for my mother. I do not want them to be overwhelmed or to feel any guilt about my care, my contentment, or my happiness. When I asked myself what I could do to make it a little easier for my children — when I reach my later years and possibly become help-less, I realized that there were a lot of questions that could be answered in advance. There were so many questions that I would like to have asked my mother. But that was never to be. It was too late for that. When I was ready to ask the questions, she was no longer able to answer them. She had become forgetful and communication was tough. Roles reversed. She became the child and her chil-dren were making all of her decisions for her.

I had not lived in my mother's home for many years. What were her fears? What were her opin-ions regarding her own health care? What deci-sions would she have made? What things would give her joy? These questions and others have led me to write this guide. If I cannot leave my children anything else, I do want to leave them **less guilt** and **more peace of mind**.

There are little things you might not have told you own family — things that are peculiar to you alone. I was thrilled when my mother turned to me and smiled at something I did to make her a bit more comfortable — and therefore a bit happier. I always felt, however, that there was more that I could have done — if only I had asked her ahead of time. Maybe, if she had left a book like this for her children, my sisters and I would have lived with less guilt and stress.

It is too late for my mother. But it is not too late for my children. I am writing this book for them, and I am writing it for all other individuals who want to help guide their future caregivers and anyone who cares.

CAVEAT

Do not assume people know
these things about you.

Do not assume that they
will remember.

TELL THEM!

As Garth Wood wrote in **The Myth of Neurosis:
Overcoming the Illness Excuse**:

*"…When the old person gives up his job and his role, his
strife and his struggle, he is frequently unable to replace
it with something of value. As he does less, his self-
respect declines and his confidence in himself fails …. If,*

however, the old person has retained his activity and interests, striving day after day to acquire new skills or perfect old ones, constantly fighting to overcome any physical deficiency resulting from the aging process, then his self-respect and self-confidence will increase ....
By being interested he becomes interesting and he need never become 'old' in the traditional sense."

INTRODUCTION

*C*AREGIVERS need guidelines on how to comfort a loved one. When individuals become our caregivers, they should have *our* guidelines available to them. We all worry about wills, funerals, and leaving finances in order — for **after we die.** This book is focused on lessening pain and stress when we are older, sometimes helpless, but *still alive*!

Therefore, this book has two audiences or sets of possible readers:

🐚   The first set constitutes those of us who recognize that we are, in fact, getting older — and that it is possible that we will one day be older, forgetful, infirm, unable to communicate feelings and desires, and/or ineffective in seeing to it that we get what we need.

🐚   The second set is made up of people who will care for us. If we are lucky, we can predict who those people will be and we can pass this book on to them. If we are lucky, they will be the people who love us — our children, other family members, or very close friends.

This book is designed to be filled out by the individual for whom future care is intended and then handed over to your future caregivers. This book is a person's chance to direct not only the care they will receive, but the "who's, what's, when's where's and how's" of his or her daily life.

Maybe it is not comfortable for you to discuss this with your caregivers. Maybe it is not comfortable for them either. Maybe you cannot even tell them you have prepared this book for their use. You can, however, leave it with important papers, on your desk, where you stash your unpaid bills, or under your address book. In other words, you can leave it where they are bound to find it when suddenly there is a need to take care of you and handle your affairs. Either way, they will have it and be able to be guided by **your wishes**.

If you are one of the lucky individuals who can discuss your wishes with your future care-givers, this book can help open all kinds of doors. If possible give it to your future caregiver now. Ask them to become familiar with it. Invite them to ask you questions. Invite them to make notes in it. Remember: this is a living document in more ways than one.

The guide is divided into eleven parts. I have made every effort to anticipate all the categories that affect our lives — not merely the big decisions, but all the little things that enhance the quality of each day.

Because this is a tool that I too will be using and filling out for my own children, there are places throughout the book where I have jumped right in and provided you, the reader, with sample answers. These are my answers for *my* children. It is there to give you an idea of the scope or detail you may wish to provide in your own responses to your future caregivers. Your responses will certainly be your own.

At the end of the eleven parts, I have added an extra chapter. To supplement the specific guidlines you provide your caregivers, I offer some general guidance that can help all of our future caregivers.

Following this final chapter, there is a section called "Notes." This contains a section of the blank pages that I promised earlier. I am sure you will think of categories that I've not included, and apply to you and your own special needs and requests. You might simply need additional space to complete comments from an earlier chapter. Make these pages your very own.

And finally, I ask that you consider writing to me and sharing your own thoughts on how the guide can be enhanced. If you have topics that you feel are important and were left out of this edition, I'd appreciate you sharing your ideas with me. I would like to improve upon this original concept and make the guide valuable to future generations.

— **Dee Marrella**

You can reach Dee at address supplied on the final page of this book.

PUBLISHER'S COMMENT

*W*HEN WE'RE YOUNG, there seems no limit, no end to life. Most of us spend very little of our lives contemplating old age or pending illness. When mid-life hits us, the majority of us are shocked. It seems like only yesterday that I went to bed a vibrant eighteen-year-old and after a fairly restful night I awoke to be fifty. That can be very shocking.

For any of us who have seen a parent become incapacitated, it can be a real education. When that illness leads to a nursing home or hospitalization or prolonged home care, the "education" can become a nightmare for all concerned. It doesn't have to be that way, but for many it is. Nerves that were once strong become frayed. Minds that were once sharp as tacks become incapable of even short-term memory. Muscles weaken. Conversations become laborious. Everyone is impacted.

For those taking on the role of caregivers, the responsibilities can become overwhelming. While much has changed in the past twenty years, when it comes to survival rates and use of life-sustaining drugs and machines, the process of caring for a loved one who once was perhaps your own source of strength, can be challenging beyond belief. Sometimes it isn't merely a matter of money. Money cannot always guarantee that the care-giving process will be smooth and event free. Nothing can guarantee a smooth experience.

With that said, it is possible for the well-intended individual who can look, with understanding, into the future to help those who will become their caregivers — help them to be prepared for some (surely not all) of the contingent events that may befall them. If one takes the time now — before something happens to drastically change their lives — it is possible that they — YOU — can provide critically important information and data to your future caregivers and assist them in providing a more positive and rewarding experience.

This guidebook was created by an individual who has gone through the care-giving process — someone who learned much from her experience. It is through her experience, recognizing the successes and the failures, and through the influence of others that she has written this tool. If you are the individual filling out the pages of this guide, I know that your future caregivers will appreciate your efforts. If you are acquiring this book for someone else, rest assured that you are giving them something that they and their caregivers will find extremely valuable.

During the final stages of preparing this book for the printer, the author sent me a copy of an article she had read in *The Philadelphia Inquirer*. After reading it, I contacted the author and obtained his permission to reprint it here. My thanks goes out to Dan Gottlieb, a clinical psychologist from Philadelphia, Pennsylvania for his wonderful article entitled **A father, a son, and a vacation that won't be forgotten.**

Vacation is over and I am a little sad. That's not news. Everyone is a little sad after vacation. I am not sad about returning to work, I am sad about leaving my vacation roommate. For the past month, I have been living with my 88-year-old father.

Several years ago I never would have believed such a time could be filled with joy. That's because when my mother died in January 1998, my father was consumed with grief. After 56 years of being in a loving marriage, it was almost a year before he could hear her name without crying. His grief was raw and deep. But something good came out of the process. He and I were always close, but after her death we became even closer. For the first time in our relationship, he would share his sadness, regret and fear of the future.

As his grief diminished, he met a "friend," whom he would occasionally take to dinner. His friend became much more than that, and, in our daily phone conversations, he would excitedly talk about his new relationship and his redis-covered libido! For the first time in years, he was animated and happy. One day about a year ago, while we were driving together, he got frustrated and said: "I don't even know why I am pursuing this relationship. I can't have sex any-way." I thought that, after 55 years, it was time to have "the talk." It was both awkward and tender as a paralyzed son talked to a father who'd had his prostate removed about what it really means to have sex. We talked about some of the many ways people find pleasure and love each other.

Despite his joy, I had watched with sadness and con-cern as his 88 years began to take their toll on his body. Although his mind remained clear, his vision and hearing both diminished and he developed a heart condition. Maybe that's what got me thinking about my dream.

Ever since I graduated from Atlantic City High School in 1964, I have dreamed about returning to the Shore for the summer. Despite my father's advancing age, I probably would have postponed my dream a few more years. But several months ago I learned that a friend of mine had died. This was a fellow quadriplegic — a man my age who had gone through rehabilitation with me. When his daughter informed me of his death, she said: "After 20 years as a quadriplegic, his body just gave out." I have been a quadriplegic for 22 years.

Later that day, I remembered a bumper sticker someone sent me years ago: "Don't postpone joy." So I called my father, who still lives in Atlantic City, and asked him how he felt about making his apartment wheelchair-accessible and spending the month of July with me. He was thrilled.

As the time drew closer, he grew more excited and I grew more concerned. He told me he was intending to cancel all his plans for the month so we could be together. I told him that although I wanted to spend time with him, I also needed time alone. I worried that his lifestyle had become restricted and the month would be depressing.

In the beginning of July, I arrived to discover that my concerns about his being intrusive on my time were unfounded. His relationship with his friend didn't last very long, but his libido sure did! Now he has other "friends." I watched with delight as he went out for various meals and activities with different friends while I stayed home or went to the movies.

Over the course of the month we became roommates in every sense of the word. I teased him about his memory and he teased me when I left the screen door open and I hollered at him for being too rigid about time. We shared jokes, lunches, and we worried about each other.

But mostly we just talked. At the time, it seemed like what we talked about was not very important — where he was going to dinner, what television shows he liked, how he dealt with his insomnia, and various other chronic problems. But as I look back on those talks I realize that he was telling me about his life — the same way I told him about my life when I was in college.

Now I know that he religiously watches Jeopardy! When he is not out on a date. And that his brother calls at exactly 9 every morning. I know that he loves to read murder mysteries and always reads the last page first to make sure it has a happy ending. Little bits of information that seem trivial. As I leave the apartment, I have a picture of a day in his life. I also have other pictures etched in my memory from this vacation. I watched as he sat in his lounge chair holding his book 12 inches from his face, moving his head from side to side, drinking in each line. I watched as he slept in that same chair with the book in his lap. I watched as he sometimes stared out the window, lost in his own thoughts, his face reflecting whether he was thinking about his past or his future.

And I watched the animation as he spoke on the phone to one of his friends, and his loud laughter when he heard something funny or ribald. Each one of these observations felt like a snapshot in my mind that I pray will not fade when his chair is empty.

Best vacation I ever had.

Thanks, Dad.

After the first time I read Dan's story, it brought back one thought and mental flash back to my own father — to my mother — my grandparents. Suddenly the purpose of Dee Marrella's guidebook became even more crystal clear. It is all of those great old stories, those fleeting memories and mental photographs that we wish we could see first-hand again. Where did all of those tons of memories go? Why can't I recall as much as I wish I could? Oh how painful it can be to want to recall those moments — and you can't.

That is why this guidebook is so important. It provides the mental kick-in-the-pants that we need to spill out on paper the thoughts and memories that our caregivers will be able to make use of at some later time and place. Here is our opportunity to speak in the future — perhaps when we cannot speak at all.

I hope that each one of you who picks up this book is inspired to put down in writing those seemingly-insignificant facts and bits of data about yourself that one day may make all the difference in the world to your caregivers — and to YOU.

— **Dennis McClellan**

January 1, 2002

PART I
General Instructions

**Sometimes life has a way of
putting us on our backs in order
to force us to look up.**

Charles L. Allen

SUGGESTIONS

1. Complete this book **NOW** — not later.

2. Place this guide where future caregivers can easily find it.

3. Update the contents once a year, if possible. (Very few things will change.)

4. Remember to tell your caregivers that they are all just human beings. If they have done all they can to love you, comfort you, and help you maintain your *dignity* — **they can not do more**.

A LETTER TO MY FUTURE CAREGIVERS

*T*HE FOLLOWING LETTER WAS written to my three daughters, Tammy, Lani and Robin. I wrote it with love from the bottom of my heart. It will go in my personal guide to my caregivers.

Write a similar letter now, while you are able to convey your true feelings. Do not worry about spelling or grammar. Just say what is in your heart. It will mean so much later on. Just do it!

The letter begins on the following page …

Dear Tammy, Lani and Robin,

One of my deepest fears is the thought of one day growing old and helpless. I pray that God takes me first. However, there is a strong possibility that He will not. In that case, I want to make the burden of your caring for me as easy and gentle as possible.

When Grandmom became "dead weight" and she had to enter a nursing home, I think you can remember how much it broke my heart. She always asked my sisters and me to promise never to put her into a nursing home. I promised, with sincere, loving intentions — but could not keep my promise when she was beyond my physical and mental capabilities. I never want any of you to proclaim that you would never put your mother or father in a nursing home. Sometimes it will be beyond your control. All I ask is that you research and find a home that "feels right" for me. Is the staff friendly? Do the residents look clean and content? Are there visitors around? If possible, I would like a private room. (You know how I react to bad odors, etc.) Please keep air fresheners and potpourri in my room.

When you come to visit, please don't tell me you can't stay very long. That tells me that you are there because of obligation. Truthfully, in that case, I would rather you stay away and get whatever is rushing you out of the way. Just come and see me when you can spend quality time holding my hand, talking to me and seeing that I am okay. I say all of the above with love and understanding — not with anger.

Remember that your husband and children take priority. I know what it was like juggling children's activities, meals, household necessities, husband's needs, and to worry and feel guilty about my sick mother. Remember when Grandmom Bea was in the nursing home? I was living in Pennsylvania. Your Dad and I decided that I would leave Pennsylvania every Monday morning and spend Monday and Tuesday in New Jersey with Grandmom. I would pick her up at 9:30 AM and take her back at 4 PM. Each day I would try to plan to have some of her friends meet us at the mall. This sometimes became difficult because she was 91 and most of her friends had passed away. Anyway, by Tuesday at 4 PM, when I dropped her off before heading back to PA, I was exhausted and filled with guilt about having to leave her. I never left her once when she said, "Thank you for coming. I had a nice time. I'll see you next time." She would always look depressed and would say, "Why do you always have to leave so soon?" I realized she didn't want to be where she was. She was always such an alive, active person. I would drive home crying and feeling guilty. I never want you girls to feel that way. I thank you, from the bottom of my heart, for **any quality time** you will give me in the future. Never feel guilty when you have to leave.

If I am visiting in your home, please talk to me. I may get deaf and I might have weak eyesight, but I can cope with these. I could not cope, however, with being tolerated or forgotten. I desire to be a viable member of the family. I want my grandchildren to love me and want to be around me. Laughter is such a healer. It bothers me so much to see older people sitting amongst others and just listening and not joining in. (Do they feel left out? Do they not want to interact? What makes them feel this way?)

Tammy, Lani and Robin — I want to thank you for being such wonderful daughters. You have always been there when Dad and I needed you. When you heard about Dad's heart operation, Tammy, you organized a schedule so that each of you would spend one week with me. By the end of three weeks, Dad was well on his way to recovery. Lani and Robin — remember when you got the initial call saying Dad had his heart attack? You came right to the hospital in Pennsylvania from New Jersey without packing or grabbing your purses. That shows how little you thought of yourselves at a time when you were needed.

Very often a little old lady sat in a wheelchair by the main entry to Grandmom's nursing home. I would give her a big greeting and hug each time I saw her. One day she grabbed my arm and pulled me back. She said, "I want you to promise to remember what I am going to tell you. When they put me in this nursing home, they took away my house, my car, my furniture — but they couldn't take away my memories. Go out and get as many good memories as you can."

Tammy, Lani and Robin — thank you for being such loving daughters. I have many wonderful, happy memories of times shared with you. I love you!

Mom

PS: Always help each other.

PERSONAL LETTER TO MY FUTURE CAREGIVERS

Date: _____

Dear: _____

_____

_____

_____

_____

_____

_____

_____

WHO CARES

GENERAL INSTRUCTIONS

WHO CARES

FOR MY CAREGIVERS: WHAT I HAVE LEARNED IN LIFE

*T*HE FOLLOWING LIST is offered as an example of my own personal beliefs! You should feel free to express your own outlook on life to your future caregivers on the pages that follow.

- Teach your children that respect and manners do not cost a dime — but oh how far they will take them in life.

- In large decisions in life, decide what is in your heart. Do not just think with your head.

- No one can take the place of a Mom or Dad in raising children.

🐚 Do not do anything you would not be proud to have your children do in the future. They are watching.

🐚 Raise your children to be proud of his/her faith, religion and nationality. Be an example.

🐚 A child is blessed if he/she is intelligent. If this child, however, is self-centered, selfish or disrespectful, he or she will be viewed as a failure.

🐚 Do not rush through life. Enjoy each other. Enjoy your children. Make "happy memories" together. Laugh and cry together. Cherish the time you have together. It goes by so quickly.

🐚 Instill in each other that, between family members, there should never be "measuring." Never measure: who called last; who entertained last, who got what. Be there to help in time of need. Be there to share when you can give your time. Be a "cheerleader" for each other.

- Expect respect from your children. They will thank you later.

- Do not have children you do not have time for. Raising a child properly is the hardest, but most gratifying, job in the whole world.

- Try not to build walls between your children and you. Listen when they want to talk to you. Do not slough off something that is bothering them as silly. Show them the respect and understanding they need.

- Teach your children to view all humans as equals. We are all here to live a life to its fullest. Teach them to despise hateful behavior. Teach them respect for race and religion. There is so much to gain if we all learn from and respect each other.

WHAT I HAVE
LEARNED IN LIFE
MY PERSONAL BELIEFS:

GENERAL INSTRUCTIONS

WHO CARES

PART II
Priorities for Care

Those who bring sunshine to the lives of others cannot keep it from themselves.

James M. Barrie

Address each section below as completely as possible

Note: Update this section whenever there is a change in medication, attending physicians, etc.

Physical problems I have and medications I take for them (include all prescription and across-the-counter drugs):

Allergies I have and medications I take for them (include all prescription and across-the-counter drugs):

My family history of reproductive problems (miscarriages, stillbirths, infertility, birth defects):

My family history of diseases (diabetes, cardiac, mental challenges, etc.):

_____

_____

_____

_____

_____

_____

_____

_____

_____

_____

_____

_____

MY FAVORITE PRODUCT BRANDS

Toothpaste: _____

Mouthwash: _____

Laxative: _____

Headache Remedy: _____

Vitamins:
 General Multivitamin: _____
 Vitamin C: _____
 Other: _____
 Other: _____
 Other: _____

Deodorant: _____

Perfume/Cologne/Aftershave Lotion: _____

Lipstick Color: _____

PRIORITIES FOR CARE

Makeup:

      1. _____

      2. _____

      3. _____

Hair Coloring Kit: _____

Hairspray: _____

Nail Polish: _____

Moisturizer: _____

Razor: _____

Shaving Creme: _____

Facial Hair Remover: _____

Soap: _____

Other Items: _____

_____

IF I HAD
A TERMINAL ILLNESS

_____ I would want to know.

_____ I would not want to know.

Comments on above:

_____

_____

_____

_____

_____

_____

_____

_____

Would I want you to request any hospital or doctor to keep me alive through extreme means if I were suffering?

_____ Yes   _____ No

Comments on use of life support:

_____

_____

_____

_____

_____

_____

_____

_____

_____

WHAT IS A "LIVING WILL?"

A "LIVING WILL" IS A DOCUMENT (*also known as an advanced directive*) *that states in advance of a serious illness or accident what medical treatments you want or don't want to receive. It can also be a document in which the signer requests to be allowed to die rather than be kept alive by artificial means if disabled beyond a reasonable expectation of recovery. When signed by a competent person, it can provide guidance for medical and health-care decisions (as the termination of life support or organ donation) in the event the person becomes incompetent to make such decisions.*

A simple statement could be created and signed in front of witnesses. It is recommended that two witnesses also sign the document. Those witnesses should not be direct members of your family or someone who would benefit financially in the event of your death.

NOTE: It is very important to understand that if you fail to make a living will accessible to others, it is actually or no value and become completely worthless. Copies of your living will should be (1) kept with this guide and (2) given to any member of your immediate family that you feel should have one, (3) to your primary care physician and any specialists you work with, (4) your attorney, (5) and the hospital to which you feel you would most likely be taken in case of an emergency. If you are admitted to a nursing home, make sure the administration has a copy. It wouldn't be a bad idea to carry a copy in your purse or wallet.

Always discuss any matters of a legal nature with an attorney of your choice.

"Do I want my doctors to keep me alive through artificial means if I become seriously ill or injured?"

_____ Yes   _____ No

Specifically, I _want the following to be done_:

- If my heart stops, I do ____ do not ____ want CPR (cardio-pulmonary resuscitation).

- I do ____ do not ____ want to be placed on any mechanical breathing apparatus.

- I do ____ do not ____ wish to have any blood transfusions.

- I do ____ do not ____ want any intravenous food administered.

- I do ____ do not ____ want any liquids administered intravenously.

- If I am transported to a healthcare facility and placed on life support, I do ____ do not ____ want it stopped at the directive of my representative(s).

Comments on this subject:

I Would Like to Be an Organ Donor.

_____ Yes   _____ No

Comments on Organ Donation:

_____

_____

_____

_____

_____

_____

_____

_____

_____

_____

_____

_____

Any Special Requests Regarding Organ Donation:

MY PREFERRED HEALTHCARE PROVIDERS

Physician: Name _____
Phone _____
Address _____
_____

Dentist: Name _____
Phone _____
Address _____
_____

Podiatrist: Name _____
Phone _____
Address _____
_____

Optometrist: Name_____

Phone_____

Address_____

_____

Optician: Name_____

Phone_____

Address_____

_____

Pharmacy: Name_____

Phone_____

Address_____

_____

Hospital: Name_____

Phone_____

Address_____

_____

Other: Name_____

Phone_____

Address_____

_____

DOCTORS, HOSPITALS, OTHER PROFESSIONALS THAT I NEVER WANT TO GO BACK TO:

Name_____
Phone_____
Address_____

_____

Name_____
Phone_____
Address_____

_____

Name_____
Phone_____
Address_____

_____

MY THOUGHTS ON A NURSING HOME OR ALTERNATIVE LIVING FACILITY AND MY PERSONAL CARE PRIORITIES:

WHO AM I?
MY TYPICAL DAY

I think it important for any caregiver to understand what my typical day is like and how much it means that these routine activities and rituals be maintained as much as possible.

🐚   I usually wake at _____ AM.

🐚   I like eating breakfast at _____ AM.

🐚   Most mornings I enjoy: (examples: gardening, watching TV, reading newspapers)

_____

_____

_____

🐚   I like to eat my lunch at _____ AM or PM.

I enjoy an afternoon nap at _____ PM.

Most afternoons I enjoy:

_____

_____

_____

I like to eat dinner at _____ PM.

After dinner I enjoy:

_____

_____

_____

I usually get ready for bed at _____ PM.

I like to:

Read in bed _____ (yes or no)

Watch TV in bed _____ (yes or no)

Go right to sleep _____ (yes or no)

I speak on the phone daily to the following people:

Name _____

Relationship _____

Phone # _____

Name _____

Relationship _____

Phone # _____

Name _____

Relationship _____

Phone # _____

WHO AM I?
MY TALENTS AND INTERESTS

Musical Instruments I play (or played):

_____

_____

_____

_____

Singing Ability:

_____

_____

_____

_____

_____

Acting Ability:

_____

_____

_____

_____

Other Talents/Skills:

_____

_____

_____

_____

Hobbies:

_____

_____

_____

_____

WHO AM I?

MILTARY HISTORY(if applicable)

 I served in the:

_____ Army

_____ Navy

_____ Marines

_____ Merchant Marines

 My rank at discharge was:

_____

 My discharge date was (day, month, year):

_____

My discharge papers are filed (location):

I belong to the following veterans' organizations:

I am receiving the following pension or military disability benefits:

Any survivor benefits (list if "yes"):

PART III
My Preferences

Always be a little kinder than necessary.

James M. Barrie

EXAMPLES OF FOOD I ENJOY:

For Breakfast:

For Lunch:

For Dinner:

Foods I love and would eat at any time:

Foods I *absolutely hate* and would never eat:

Foods I am allergic to:

My favorite snack foods include:

My favorite soups are:

_____

_____

_____

My favorite salads and dressings include:

_____

_____

_____

My favorite entrees are:

_____

_____

_____

My favorite:

Candy: _____

_____

Cake: _____

_____

MY PREFERENCES

Pie: _____

_____

Ice Cream: _____

_____

When you have me in your home, here are some recipes that I really enjoy: (Write in complete recipes that you've created or make regularly, or make reference to recipes that are familiar to family members.)

_____

_____

_____

_____

_____

_____

_____

_____

WHO CARES

MY PREFERENCES

WHO CARES

MY CLOTHING SIZES

Female

_____ Dress
_____ Blouse
_____ Slacks
_____ Outer Coat
_____ Sweater
_____ Shoes
_____ Stockings
_____ Pajamas
_____ Nightgown
_____ Slippers
_____ Housecoat
_____ Slips
_____ Underpants
_____ Bras

Male

_____ Suit
_____ Shirt
_____ Trousers
_____ Outer Coat
_____ Sweater
_____ Shoes
_____ Socks
_____ Pajamas

_____ Slippers
_____ Robe
_____ Underwear
    ____ T-Shirts
         Shorts
    ____ Boxer
    ____ Briefs

WHERE TO FIND THINGS IN MY HOUSE/APARTMENT:

Medication(s)

Extra eye glasses:

Dentures:

Hearing Aid:

Walker:

Folding Wheelchair:

Insulin Equipment:

Other:

Bedtime clothing I feel most comfortable wearing (Put in order of favorites — "1" being your favorite):

_____ Nightgown
_____ Pajamas
_____ Underwear
_____ Other

My Favorite Bed Pillow: (Check one)

_____ Soft
_____ Medium
_____ Hard

I like to take: (Check one)

_____ Showers
_____ Baths

Comments on Above:

_____

_____

_____

Clothes I am most comfortable in:

_____

_____

_____

_____

_____

_____

_____

Clothes I do not like to wear:

_____

_____

_____

_____

_____

My favorite colors to wear:

_____

_____

_____

_____

_____

_____

Three favorite outfits I like to wear:

1. _____

_____

_____

2. _____

_____

_____

3. _____

_____

_____

In a nursing home, you are given one small closet (as a rule) and one dresser. What would you choose to put in these places if you had to sort through all your clothes, jewelry, books, etc. today?

What would you want on the walls of your room? (Include favorite family picture, a favorite clock, etc.) And where are these items found in your current home or apartment?

Are there any religious items that you want to always have near you? Please list and identify where they can be located.

Types of TV shows I enjoy:

Types of TV shows that I do not enjoy:

Newspapers and Magazines I enjoy reading:

Favorite movies and videos I enjoy viewing:

My favorite authors:

My favorite religious scriptures, meditations, readings:

Card games I enjoy:

Board games I enjoy:

Favorite singers:

MY PREFERENCES

Favorite movie stars:

_____

_____

_____

_____

_____

Favorite TV stars:

_____

_____

_____

_____

_____

_____

Favorite TV channels and shows:

Radio programs I enjoy:

Radio programs I do not enjoy:

Sports I like to watch:

Sport   **Favorite Team**

Ways I like to relax:

Music I enjoy listening to:

Music that gives me a headache:

MY PREFERENCES

Do you like to be around small children?

_____

_____

_____

_____

_____

_____

_____

Do you like to be around pets?

_____ Yes   _____ No

Dogs   _____

Cats   _____

Other   _____

CARING FOR MY PETS
IN A TIME OF EMERGENCY

Type of pet: _____

Name of pet: _____

Veterinarian: Name _____

Phone _____

Address _____

_____

Pet Groomer: Name _____

Phone _____

Address _____

_____

Kennel: Name _____

Phone _____

Address _____

_____

Name and telephone number of individual who
could **care for pet temporarily:**

Name_____

Phone_____

Address_____

_____

Brand of General Pet Food:

Dry_____

_____

Wet_____

_____

Brand of Biscuits:_____

Brand of Special Treats:_____

Exercise habits:_____

_____

_____

Where he/she prefers to sleep:_____

_____

_____

Would you like your pet to visit you if possible?

_____ Yes   _____ No

**Arrangements for permanent care for my pet —
to assure that my pet is loved and properly
cared for:**

_____

_____

_____

_____

_____

_____

_____

_____

_____

_____

_____

_____

PLACES I LIKE TO VISIT

Where I like to go for drives in the car:

For breakfast:

For lunch:

For dinner:

For sightseeing:

FUNERAL ARRANGEMENTS THAT I PREFER

I would like to be:

Buried
Location _____
City / State _____

Cremated
Location _____
City / State _____

Note: if any prior arrangements have been made, where can those documents be located, including plans for ashes if cremated:

_____

_____

_____

I would like to wear the color(s):

_____

_____

_____

I would like this church/temple/place of worship to be used for the ceremony (name of location, city):

Location _____

City / State _____

_____

I would like this Priest, Rabbi, Clergyman to preside over the ceremony:

Name _____

Phone _____

Address _____

_____

I would like the following music played at the place of worship:

I would like these prayers said at my funeral:

I would like to have the following inscribed on my tombstone or grave marker:

I want these items placed in the coffin with me:

I would prefer "at the viewing":

_____ An open casket _____ A closed casket

My parents are buried (location, city):

Location _____

City / State _____

PART IV
Who Am I?

The only gift is a portion of thyself.

Ralph Waldo Emerson

WHO AM I?

What are my innermost feelings about myself? What are the things about myself that I like and dislike? And what do I like and dislike about the world around me?

Keep in mind that you will have your own feelings to write down. It is also important to note that there is no set number of responses, and no response is "right" or "wrong." The following are the authors examples:

🐾 *I am very "thin skinned." My feelings can get hurt very easily. Because I am this way, I try to "feel" for others and not offend them.*

🐾 *I believe every child should get a fine education. Equally important, however, I believe* every child should be taught the importance of manners and honesty — or you, as a parent, have "shortchanged" your child.

God gave each of us special talents. It is a sin if you do not use these talents to make the world a better place.

One of the most evil things on this earth is prejudice. I try to look each person squarely in the eye and decide if I like or dislike what I see. I think it is so wrong to judge a person because of his/her color, religion or nationality. We could learn so much from each other.

I am afraid of animals. I love to watch them. I would never harm them. I was never allowed to have a pet as a child. Therefore, I keep my distance.

WHO AM I?

Here are my innermost likes and dislikes about the world around me and myself.

WHO AM I?

FEARS I HAVE?

Keep in mind that you will have your own fears to share. It is also important to note that there is no set number of fears, and no response is "right" or "wrong." The following are the author's examples.

 I am not afraid of death. I am afraid of pain and suffering. Medicate me, even if it means a shorter life

 Being treated like a child in my later life is a fear I have. Please never talk down to me or "pat me on the head." Allow me to keep my dignity.

 Make certain that I am never fed anything with a Red Sauce or Mayonnaise. I gag on both.

I am very shy. If possible, please do not let a male nurse care for me.

I fear strife in the family if Dad or I were alone and sickly. Our family has such love and closeness now. Please do not let Dad or me cause that to change. Work together. Try to keep a sense of humor. Two things have always helped me when things got really stressful with Gram: faith in God and a good laugh.

FEARS I HAVE?

_____

_____

_____

_____

_____

_____

_____

_____

_____

_____

_____

WHO AM I?

ONE SPECIFIC FEAR

One of the greatest fears people have for the future is being told that you have Alzheimer's. How can one prepare for this? How can you help your "caregivers?"

I spoke with an individual who works with Alzheimer's patients. She said that one could never predict when the patient is lucid or when the person is living in his/her past. Claudia recommended that I include this section in this guide so that the caregiver can talk and reminisce about the past with the patient. She said it would be very helpful to have an idea of what the person was like in his/her teens, 20's, 30's, etc.

Here are things I want you to know about me when I was:

IN MY TEENS:

I lived in:

- City / State _____

High School and year of graduation:

- Name / Date _____

My favorite date was (his/her name):

- _____

My favorite thing to do on a date was:

- _____

For fun, my friends and I would:

- _____

My interests and hobbies were:

- _____

Additional information:

- _____

_____

_____

_____

IN MY 20'S:

I lived in:

- City / State _____

I worked at:

- Company/Job _____

I married _____

on _____. (month/day/year)

My children's names are::

- _____ /DOB _____
- _____ /DOB _____
- _____ /DOB _____
- _____ /DOB _____

My friends included:

- _____
- _____
- _____
- _____

For fun, my friends and I would:

My interests and hobbies were:

Additional information:

IN MY 30'S:

I lived in:

👤 City / State _____

I worked at:

👤 Company/Job _____

I married _____

on _____. (month/day/year)

My children's names are::

👤 _____ /DOB _____

👤 _____ /DOB _____

👤 _____ /DOB _____

👤 _____ /DOB _____

My friends included:

👤 _____

👤 _____

👤 _____

👤 _____

WHO AM I?

For fun, my friends and I would:

My interests and hobbies were:

Additional information:

IN MY 40'S:

I lived in:

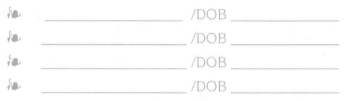 City / State _____

I worked at:

Company/Job _____

My grandchildren's names are:

_____ /DOB _____

_____ /DOB _____

_____ /DOB _____

_____ /DOB _____

My friends included:

_____

_____

_____

_____

WHO AM I?

For fun, my friends and I would:

My interests and hobbies were:

Additional information:

IN MY 50'S:

I lived in:

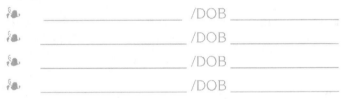 City / State _____

I worked at:

Company/Job _____

My grandchildren's names are:

_____ /DOB _____

_____ /DOB _____

_____ /DOB _____

_____ /DOB _____

My friends included:

_____

_____

_____

_____

WHO AM I?

For fun, my friends and I would:

My interests and hobbies were:

Additional information:

IN MY 60'S:

I lived in:

🐚   City / State _____

I worked at:

🐚   Company/Job _____

My grandchildren's names are:

🐚   _____ /DOB _____

🐚   _____ /DOB _____

🐚   _____ /DOB _____

🐚   _____ /DOB _____

My friends included:

🐚   _____

🐚   _____

🐚   _____

🐚   _____

For fun, my friends and I would:

My interests and hobbies were:

Additional information:

IN MY 70'S:

I lived in:

   City / State _____

I worked at:

   Company/Job _____

My grandchildren's names (Great grandchildren if there are any) are:

   _____ /DOB _____

   _____ /DOB _____

   _____ /DOB _____

   _____ /DOB _____

My friends included:

   _____

   _____

   _____

   _____

WHO AM I?

For fun, my friends and I would:

My interests and hobbies were:

Additional information:

IN MY 80'S:

I lived in:

🐾 City / State _____

My grandchildren's names (Great grandchildren if there are any) are:

🐾 _____ /DOB _____

🐾 _____ /DOB _____

🐾 _____ /DOB _____

🐾 _____ /DOB _____

My friends included:

🐾 _____

🐾 _____

🐾 _____

🐾 _____

WHO AM I?

For fun, my friends and I would:

My interests and hobbies were:

Additional information:

SPECIAL REQUESTS FOR CAREGIVERS

Keep in mind that those special requests you have for your family will be different than these. You may have more; you may have less. It's quality, not quantity that counts here.

- *I have always taught my daughters that you will never, ever find more reliable sincere friends than your own sisters or brothers.* My request: "Please do not ever close the lines of communications with one another. If something is bothering you, talk it out — together."

- *Never measure what you do for each other. Give with your whole heart when a family member is in need.*

🕊 I *would enjoy receiving* Holy Communion *when it is offered.*

🕊 *Always make faith and religion a* **family priority**.

SPECIAL REQUESTS
FOR CAREGIVERS

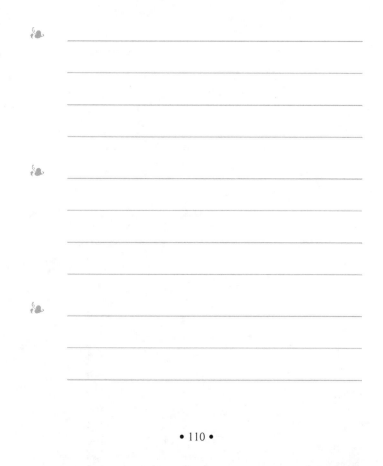

WHO AM I?

PART V
Relationships

*Whatever you do to the least of my brothers...
that you do unto me.*

Jesus

PEOPLE I LOVE AND WOULD ENJOY SEEING:

Name_____

Phone_____

Address_____

_____

Name_____

Phone_____

Address_____

_____

Name_____

Phone_____

Address_____

_____

Name_____

Phone_____

Address_____

_____

FRIENDS TO NOTIFY
IF I AM IN THE HOSPITAL:

Name_____
Phone_____
Address_____

_____

Name_____
Phone_____
Address_____

_____

Name_____
Phone_____
Address_____

_____

Name_____
Phone_____
Address_____

_____

IF ANYONE INVITED ME TO GO OUT FOR A DAY'S OUTING OR EVENING, THIS IS WHAT I WOULD REALLY ENJOY DOING:

In town:

On a trip:

PART VI
Holidays and
Religious Observances

My favorite holiday:

‮

_____

_____

_____

_____

_____

_____

_____

Why this holiday has always been so special:

‮

_____

_____

_____

_____

_____

_____

_____

What I love to do on my favorite holiday:

TRADITIONAL FAMILY HOLIDAYS

NOTE: For many people, Thanksgiving and Halloween are holidays that are observed. However, since there are many holidays throughout any given year, and considering that we all celebrate different ones in our own family structure, please fill in the ones you are most familiar with below.

Holiday_____

Family Tradition Observed_____

_____

_____

_____

_____

_____

HOLIDAYS AND RELIGIOUS OBSERVANCES

Holiday

Family Tradition Observed

Holiday

Family Tradition Observed

Holiday_____

Family Tradition Observed_____

_____

_____

_____

_____

_____

_____

Holiday_____

Family Tradition Observed:_____

_____

_____

_____

_____

_____

_____

_____

RELIGIOUS AFFILIATION

Church/Temple/Religious Facility:

_____

Address: _____

Telephone #: _____

Key Contact Names: _____

_____

_____

Describe Attendance (include time of day, seating area, and other important points):

_____

_____

_____

_____

Describe Participation (such as choir, usher, etc.):

Interesting and memorable times I would love to talk about with anyone who would listen:

I once read somewhere that the nicest things you could give an elderly loved one include:

- Your time

- Hugs and hand holding

- Time to talk, listen and reminisce about the past and happy times

Holiday vacation I enjoy the most (such as a visit to the seashore, a visit to the mountains, taking a cruise. etc.):

PART VII
Important Names

CHART OF DECENDANTS (SAMPLE FAMILY TREE)

Elvira Amendola
Mother

Daymond Delia
Father

Their Children

Theresa Delia

Delores Delia(me)
married
Leonard S. Marrella

Karen Delia

My Children

Tammy Marrella
Toso

Lani Marrella
Martin

Robin Marrella
Russo

My Grandchildren

Tory Toso
Todd Toso

Len Belotti
Roseanne Martin
Danielle Martin

Ryan Russo
Casey Russo

My Birth:
St. Joseph's Hosital
Paterson, New Jersey
December 4th, 1935

YOUR CHART OF DECENDANTS

Mother

Father

Their Children

_____ (me)

married

My Children

My Grandchildren

My Birth:

PERSONAL INFORMATION

Last Name: _____

First Name: _____

Middle Name: _____

Nickname: _____

Named After: _____

Birth Date: _____

Current Address: _____

_____

_____

Current Telephone Number: _____

EDUCATION

Elementary School

Name: _____

Location: _____

Junior High or Middle School

Name: _____

Location: _____

High School

Name: _____

Location: _____

College/University

Undergraduate:

    Location: _____

    Major: _____

    Minor: _____

    Degree Received: _____

    Honors: _____

Graduate:

    Location: _____

    Major: _____

    Minor: _____

    Degree Received: _____

CAREER — JOBS HELD

Company Name:

    Location: _____

    Job Title/Description: _____

    Years Employed There: _____

Company Name:

    Location: _____

    Job Title/Description: _____

    Years Employed There: _____

Company Name:

    Location: _____

    Job Title/Description: _____

    Years Employed There: _____

PARENTS — MOTHER

Maiden Name: _____

First Name: _____

Middle Name: _____

Birth Date: _____

Birthplace: _____

If Applicable:

Death Date: _____

Cause of Death: _____

Place of Burial: _____

Location: _____

PARENTS — FATHER

Last Name: _____

First Name: _____

Middle Name: _____

Birth Date: _____

Birthplace: _____

If Applicable:

Death Date: _____

Cause of Death: _____

Place of Burial: _____

Location: _____

CHILDREN

Full Name: _____

Date of Birth: _____

Birthplace: _____

Current Residence: _____

Full Name: _____

Date of Birth: _____

Birthplace: _____

Current Residence: _____

Full Name: _____

Date of Birth: _____

Birthplace: _____

Current Residence: _____

IMPORTANT NAMES

Full Name: _____

Date of Birth: _____

Birthplace: _____

Current Residence: _____

Full Name: _____

Date of Birth: _____

Birthplace: _____

Current Residence: _____

Full Name: _____

Date of Birth: _____

Birthplace: _____

Current Residence: _____

MEDICAL HISTORY

The following is a list of known medical conditions/major injuries that should be noted:

Name of illness/injury:

Age of occurrence: _____

Type of Treatment: _____

_____

_____

Long-term impact: _____

_____

_____

_____

Name of illness/injury:

Age of occurrence: _____

Type of Treatment: _____

_____

_____

Long-term impact: _____

_____

_____

_____

Name of illness/injury:

Age of occurrence: _____

Type of Treatment: _____

_____

_____

Long-term impact: _____

_____

_____

_____

Name of illness/injury:

Age of occurrence: _____

Type of Treatment: _____

_____

_____

Long-term impact: _____

_____

_____

_____

Name of illness/injury:

Age of occurrence: _____

Type of Treatment: _____

_____

_____

Long-term impact: _____

_____

_____

_____

IMPORTANT NAMES

Name of illness/injury:

Age of occurrence: _____

Type of Treatment: _____

_____

_____

Long-term impact: _____

_____

_____

_____

Name of illness/injury:

Age of occurrence: _____

Type of Treatment: _____

_____

_____

Long-term impact: _____

_____

_____

_____

PART VIII
Financial and
Business Affairs

MY BUSINESS AFFAIRS

Locating and understanding where important papers can be found (provide location, contact person if needed, contact phone numbers):

Will:

Name_____

Phone _____

Address _____

_____

Checking Account(s):

Name_____

Phone _____

Address _____

_____

Account Number(s) _____

Savings Account(s):

Name _____

Phone _____

Address _____

_____

Account Number(s) _____

Stock Certificates:

Name _____

Phone _____

Address _____

_____

Owner's Name _____

Name _____

Phone _____

Address _____

_____

Owner's Name _____

WHO CARES

Name_____

Phone_____

Address_____

_____

Owner's Name_____

Name_____

Phone_____

Address_____

_____

Owner's Name_____

Name_____

Phone_____

Address_____

_____

Owner's Name_____

Bonds:

Name

Phone

Address

Owner's Name

Insurance Policies:

Name

Phone

Address

Policy Number

Name

Phone

Address

Policy Number

Name _____

Phone _____

Address _____

_____

Policy Number _____

Name _____

Phone _____

Address _____

_____

Policy Number _____

Special Collections
(i.e., stamps, coins, other collectables):

Item Name: _____

Name _____

Phone _____

Address _____

_____

DISTRIBUTION OF ASSETS

NOTE: your will is the single best tool for delineating what items of value are to be distributed to which individual(s). The list below can serve as a backup tool. List here "Item" and name(s) of recipients. Be as specific as you can.

How I would like my loved ones to divide my furnishings, jewelry, etc.:

IMPORTANT NAMES AND PHONE NUMBERS

Important Names and Phone Numbers (this list includes individuals you deal with both personally and for business):

Bank

Name

Phone

Address

List all account numbers

Financial Planner

Name

Phone

Address

Lawyer

Name

Phone

Address

Accountant

Name

Phone

Address

Broker

Name

Phone

Address

Money Market Fund

Name

Phone

Address

Account Number(s)

Funeral Home

Name

Phone

Address

Safety Deposit Box/Keys

Name

Phone

Address

Box Number

Comments:

WHERE TO LOCATE IMPORTANT PAPERS:

CREDIT CARDS:

Visa:

Account # _____

MasterCard:

Account # _____

Discover:

Account # _____

American Express:

Account # _____

Other Credit Cards:

Account #

Location/Comments:

Bank Account Books:

Location/Comments:

Rental Property Payment Books:

Location/Comments:

Other Financial Records:

Location/Comments:_____

_____

_____

_____

_____

IMPORTANT KEYS:

Keys to House/Apartment:

Location/Comments: _____

_____

Keys to Car(s):

Location/Comments: _____

_____

Other Important Keys:

Location/Comments: _____

_____

WILL:

Two people with copies of my will:

Name

Address

Phone #

Name

Address

Phone #

POWERS OF ATTORNEY

Two people with Powers of Attorney:

Name

Address

Phone #

Name

Address

Phone #

BIRTH CERTFICATE:

Two people with copies of my birth certificate:

Name _____

Address _____

Phone # _____

Name _____

Address _____

Phone # _____

MY SOCIAL SECURITY #:

_____

INSURANCE POLICIES:

Name of Insurance Company _____

Insurance Company Phone # _____

Policy # _____

Address of Company _____

_____

Location of Policy _____

FINANCIAL AND BUSINESS AFFAIRS

Name of Insurance Company _____

Insurance Company Phone # _____

Policy # _____

Address of Company _____

_____

Location of Policy _____

Name of Insurance Company _____

Insurance Company Phone # _____

Policy # _____

Address of Company _____

_____

Location of Policy _____

Cash or Long Term Care Policy that I have to cover nursing home costs:

Name of Policy _____

Policy # _____

Address of Carrier _____

Location of Policy _____

Name of Policy _____

Policy # _____

Address of Carrier _____

Location of Policy _____

Name of Policy _____

Policy # _____

Address of Carrier _____

Location of Policy _____

List of Personal Assets:

Name of Item _____

Location of Item _____

Appraisal _____

Location of Appraisal _____

Name of Item _____

Location of Item _____

Appraisal _____

Location of Appraisal _____

Name of Item _____

Location of Item _____

Appraisal _____

Location of Appraisal _____

Name of Item _____

Location of Item _____

Appraisal _____

Location of Appraisal _____

Pensions and Retirement Accounts:

Title of Pension Plan/Retirement Account:

_____

Account Number: _____

Location: _____

_____

Title of Pension Plan/Retirement Account:

_____

Account Number: _____

Location: _____

_____

Title of Pension Plan/Retirement Account:

_____

Account Number: _____

Location: _____

_____

Home:

Address: _____

Purchase Price: _____

Current Value: _____

Date of last appraisal: _____

Location of Deed(s): _____

Automobile(s):

Make/Model: _____

Year: _____

Location of Title: _____

Make/Model: _____

Year: _____

Location of Title: _____

Make/Model: _____

Year: _____

Location of Title: _____

Other Assets:

Furs

Comments: _____

_____

_____

Jewelry

Comments: _____

_____

_____

Antiques

Comments: _____

_____

_____

Stamps:

Comments: _____

_____

_____

FINANCIAL AND BUSINESS AFFAIRS

Coins:

Comments: _____

_____

_____

Other:

Comments: _____

_____

_____

_____

_____

_____

_____

_____

_____

_____

_____

_____

Any Debts Owed:

Type: _____

Name to be paid: _____

Address: _____

Phone # _____

Type: _____

Name to be paid: _____

Address: _____

Phone # _____

Type: _____

Name to be paid: _____

Address: _____

Phone # _____

Type: _____

Name to be paid: _____

Address: _____

Phone # _____

PART IX

Life's Lessons

*What I have learned in life and
would like to pass on to my loved ones.*

"My children are coming today. They mean well, but they worry. They think I should have a railing in the hall, a telephone in the kitchen. They want someone to come in when I take a bath. They don't really like my living alone. Help me to be grateful for their concern. And help them to understand that I have to do what I can as long as I can. They're right when they say there are risks. I might fall. I might leave the stove on. But there is no challenge, no possibility of triumph, no real aliveness without risk. When they were young and rode bicycles and climbed trees and went away to camp, I was terrified, but I let them go. Because to hold them would have been to hurt them. Now roles are reversed. Help them to see. Keep me from being grim or stubborn about it. But don't let them smother me."

— **Elise Maclay,** St. Cloud Visitor

REGRETS IN MY LIFE

If I had to do it all over again…

Regrets:

Special interests I wish I had pursued:

What is really important in life:

QUESTIONS ASKED OF SEVERAL PEOPLE
What Have You Learned Over Your Lifetime?

*Note: Most of the lessons learned (and remembered) listed below involve people not "things."

- I've learned that I like my teacher because she cries when we sing *Silent Night*.

  —Age 6

- I've learned that our dog doesn't want to eat my broccoli either. —Age 7

🐚 I've learned that just when I get my room the way I like it; Mom makes me clean it up again. — Age 12

🐚 I've learned that if you want to cheer yourself up; you should try cheering someone else up. — Age 14

🐚 I've learned that although it's hard to admit it, I'm secretly glad my parents are strict with me. — Age 15

🐚 I've learned that silent company is often more healing than words of advice.
— Age 24

🐚 I've learned that brushing my child's hair is one of life's great pleasures. — Age 26

🍂 I've learned that there are people who love you dearly but just don't know how to show it. — Age 42

🍂 I've learned that you can make someone's day by simply sending them a little note. — Age 44

🍂 I've learned that children and grandparents are natural allies. — Age 47

🍂 I've learned that no matter what happens, or how bad it seems today, life goes on, and it will be better tomorrow. — Age 48

🍂 I've learned that singing *Amazing Grace* can lift my spirits for hours. — Age 49

I've learned that you can tell a lot about a man by the way he handles these three things: a rainy day, lost luggage and tangled Christmas tree lights.

— Age 52

I've learned that regardless of your relationship with your parents, you miss them terribly after they die.

— Age 53

I've learned that making a living is not the same thing as making a life.

— Age 58

I've learned that life sometimes gives you a second chance.

— Age 62

I've learned that if you pursue happiness, it will elude you. But if you focus on your family, the needs of others, your work, meeting new people, and doing the very best you can, happiness will find you. — Age 65

I've learned that whenever I decide something with kindness, I usually make the right decision. — Age 66

I've learned that everyone can use a prayer. — Age 72

I've learned that it pays to believe in miracles. And to tell the truth, I've seen several. — Age 75

I've learned that even when I have pains, I don't have to be one. — Age 82

I've learned that every day you should reach out and touch someone. People love a human touch, holding hands, a warm hug, or just a friendly pat on the back. — Age 85

I've learned that I still have a lot to learn. — Age 92

I've learned that you should pass this on to someone you care about. Sometimes they just need a little something to make them smile. — Ageless

— Anonymous

A MESSAGE TO THE READER

Dear Reader:

Hopefully, this guidebook will give you some ideas as to what lies ahead as you get older and dependent upon other human beings.

In this guide, I spoke of the nursing home and the impact it had on me. I have observed and have learned. I have met some warm, wonderful residents. They would prefer being home, but they know (most of them, that is) that they need additional help. I have also seen many unhappy, ornery older residents. I truly believe that people do not change that much. If he/she was unfriendly and hateful as a young person, that is the same type of person he/she will be as an older person, at home or in a nursing home.

I have written the following story based on a certain patient I met at a nursing home. Perhaps this story will drive home the point that you, as an independent, vital person must **evaluate your life NOW**. Where is your life heading? Will your later life be filled with love or loneliness? Are you taking time to nurture relationships? I contend, while you are young you must plan for your monetary security. But — and this is a big "BUT" — not at the expense of family and friends. Stay in contact and enjoy the important people in your life. It is not a sin to desire wealth — but it is pitiful when it means you have no time to love and enjoy family and friends.

A WASTED LIFE

My God, I must be having a nightmare! What am I doing here? Who are these strangers? When did this happen to me? I was always in control of my own life. What went wrong? I don't like some of these awful odors!

I hear myself yelling, "Nurse! Nurse! Help me!" A pretty person in a white uniform walks in and tells me to stop yelling. I want to know where I am. She pats me on the shoulder and says that I am in the "Nursing Home." She tells me everything is going to be all right and that I will soon get used to where I am. I don't want to get used to where I am! I don't want to get used to this place! She tells me to relax. She will be right back to wash and dress me. I wait and wait. I doze off. I awaken and try to clear my head. I try to remember how I got here.

I remember tripping over a rug in my study and falling. I lay there in pain all night. I got cold and yelled. No one heard me. I lived alone. I couldn't reach the phone. I was divorced and not close to my children. I knew no one would be phoning to see how I was. I passed out. When I awakened I was in the hospital with a broken hip. My cleaning woman had found me in the morning and had called an ambulance. From the hospital, I was brought here.

I look around my room and see a wheelchair. Will I sit in it for the rest of my life? I hear a lot of activity and a lot of announcements. I lay there thinking — thinking — always thinking. Thinking makes me "clammy" all over. I don't want to think. People used to tell me how much they needed faith in their lives. Not me. I was in control and doing just fine. Look at me now. Who is in control now?

Would God listen and forgive my self-centered, self-ish life? Is it too late? Where is my family? Why hasn't anyone called?

What am I good for anymore? Nobody needs me. How "self-important" am I now? When I was young, I swore I would someday live in a beautiful home, have expensive cars and lots of money. I wanted the whole package. But where did all the power and money get me? All my "things" are now left behind. None of the prestige and wealth I craved can comfort me now. How stupid I was to crave for — what? I look around my room. I see a wheelchair, a dresser, a nightstand, a small TV, a chair, a sink, and a closet. That's it for "things" for me from now on. I look at the open doorway, hoping to see one familiar face. Why in heaven would I expect love and attention now? I never took time to give it.

Sure I had a wife and family, but they came second to my career. How could my children expect me to get away from work to see their plays and games? I was the "breadwinner!" How could they expect me to be home on time for dinner at night? I was the "breadwinner!" How could my wife not understand when I had to frequently cancel out on social engagements? I was the "breadwinner!" As a husband and father, I was out making a living. A wife and mother took care of the home and children. When did it happen? When did my wife and children finally leave me out of their lives? All of a sudden, I wasn't asked to join in much anymore. Their lives went on without me. Weren't they impressed with my success and power at work?

Throughout my life, I wanted to prove that I had made it. I wanted to be seen at the right places with the right people. Where are all these people — the "right people" — now? I am beginning to realize who the "right people" really were. My kind cleaning woman had so little yet managed to tolerate my tirades and remain patient. My neighbor, who was from another country and tried so hard to be my friend, but I wasn't interested. What could he do for me? Wrong nationality. Wrong profession. Now I realize that he was trying to give me something from his heart — his time and his attention. There was no ulterior motive. How I would love his friendship now! I looked down on so many people. I was so prejudiced and judgmental. It made me feel good to think that I was better than others — richer, smarter, right image. Better! Better! Better! Am I *better* now? A lonely, scared old man? If only I could go back. How much I lost in life by not getting to know so many nice people who crossed my path. Why did I let so much hate and prejudice get in my way? What a waste!

I'm sitting in the doorway of my room now just watching people. I see Joan — a crippled, bent over, old lady who tries so hard to smile and be *pleasant. Doesn't she know where she is? Why is it some people can adjust and make almost any situation **"okay?"** Joan has constant visitors. Her family visits often. People passing by her stop and give her a smile and a hug. Now who is wealthier? Me, with lots of money and almost no personal contact? Or Joan who is surrounded by sincere warmth from caring people? I can't buy that. I can't force that.*

Why did I feel I always had to compete with my brother as an adult? Growing up we had been very close. Later on, I had little time for anything but work. We grew apart. Bob moved out of state. I heard his wife needed dental work and couldn't afford it. I heard he and his wife worked to make ends meet. I had heard my nieces and nephews worked their way through college. Why didn't I step in and help? Did I feel a little superior seeing them struggle? Did I want to prove my success by waiting for him to come to me and ask for help? Little did I know I was measuring my success against his only by the total in my bank account. How short-sighted! I didn't see how many hours per day my brother put aside to attend his children's games and school activities. I never saw them all together, each night at dinner, laughing and sharing the day's events. I never saw the nights Bob and Mary were content being together watching TV. I hear he has a loving, growing family with a lot of happy memories surrounding him. Who won the "competition" between brothers? Who ended up wealthier?

I wonder where my children are. Do they ever speak lovingly of me? Will they ever come to see me? Why hasn't anyone called? I always threatened them that at any point I could take them out of my will. Don't they care anymore? Why hasn't anyone called? Please God, don't let me die a lonely, frightened old man. Oh God, what have I done to myself?

GENERAL GUIDANCE FOR CAREGIVERS

I *do pray that when I am elderly…*

- I will be kept clean.

- I will be fed nutritious meals.

- I will be helped to keep my dignity as much as possible.

- I will obtain necessary medical care.

- I will not be treated as though I am already dead. I hope I will have the opportunity to continue to be around things I love — family, friends, jokes, music, movies, and good food until the day I do die!!

- I hope to be remembered for the love and support I tried to give to my family and friends. To be loved in return is to have true wealth.

While I am still "rational," I do realize that later on...

- You cannot be with me 24 hours a day.

- You must go on with your life.

- You love me and will try to do your best to help keep me comfortable.

- At times, you will feel anger and guilt when I thrash out in frustration. I am not angry with you. I am angry and frustrated that I have become helpless and older.

- You did not make me older or sick.

- You must take care of your family and yourself. Don't feel guilty when you cannot be with me. Go on with your life.

Signed: _____

(Your signature here)

NOTE TO
MY CAREGIVERS
Things I learned
When I was a Caregiver

SINCE YOU ARE THE ONE who will be in need of care in the future, feel free to add anything you feel appropriate. If you disagree with something, cross it out. This guide must become "your guide."

If you have brothers or sisters, **do not** expect every one of them to take care of your parent in the same way. Each person has to live with his/her own decisions. Each should pretend he/she is **an only child**. Do not compare notes about what each one is doing or not doing. It only leads to anger, family strife and illness. You do what you can — with love.

Do not look for praise or condemnation. It is to God that you have to answer. If you truly believe you are doing your share to help care and give your loved one love and kindness, so be it.

It is so much easier to care for a loved one when everyone **cooperates**. Talk together. Plan together. Just don't compare!

When you visit an elderly person, give him/her your **undivided attention**. Do not always look rushed and frustrated. Sometime you might be the only visitor he/she sees for days. A hug, kiss and sincere smile means so much. Sit close and hold his/her hand. **Show** the love you feel.

Before each visit, take a minute to visualize yourself in the condition and environment. What would be **your** physical and emotional needs?

Do not **talk down** to the person for whom you are providing care.

Take the person out of their environment as much as possible. Let him/her feel alive. A mall is a great place to go. (People to watch, varieties of food, accommodations for wheelchairs, and bathrooms are accessible.) Such small "outings" will let the person know his/her "confinement" will not be continuous.

If possible, bring a favorite food when you visit. (I find that elderly people talk among themselves about food, ailments and constipation! Wouldn't you rather they talked about food?) For an extra special treat, set a pretty table with flowers, etc. Bring an up-to-date album to show the latest family pictures.

I always try to remember what a friend, Sister Jo Anne, said to me. "Dee, you did not make your mother old, and you did not make her sick. You can love her and try to make her life as comfortable as possible, but you cannot make her young and happy. You are not God."

Carry a comb, makeup, nail polish, etc. with you if you are visiting an elderly female. My Mother loved to look nice like we all do. Remember that he/she is elderly, not dead! If the person you are visiting is male, why not surprise him with his favorite aftershave or cologne?

Before I would leave, I always handed my Mom a newspaper, magazine or something I knew she enjoyed. That way, she had something to look forward to when I left. Leave with a big hug and a promise to return.

Each time I would leave, I told my Mom something she could look forward to when I came back. "Mom, Tuesday we will visit Peggy. Mom, I am bringing Alice to visit with you on Thursday. Mom, I am taking you to the shore on Monday and Tuesday." Everyone needs a reason to go on living.

Someone once told me to put cotton in my ears, Vaseline on my glasses, and heavy gloves on my hands and combat boots on my feet. This will give you some idea of how an elderly person sees, hears, and feels.

Remember that we are all aging. Treat your loved one the way you would want to be treated.

Do not kid yourself into thinking your own children are not watching. They are observing how lovingly you treat your Mom and Dad or other family members. More often than not, that is the way you will be treated someday.

Be fair, loving, kind, and compassionate. Keep calm, but stay in control.

Signed: _____

(Your signature here)

IDEAS AND GIFTS TO HELP THE ELDERLY

- To pay bills or run errands for your care recipient, have him/her put all bills and list of needs into one box. You can pick these up when you visit.

- Leave a few dollars so that a pizza can be ordered or some other special treat. (Some patients met as a group and did this weekly.)

- If the person is in a wheelchair, clip a portable digital phone to the chair. (Purchase one that has 1-button-dialing for often-used numbers.)

- Purchase a clock with large numerals for the wall.

- Purchase a calendar with large squares and fill in important family dates: birthdays, anniversaries, etc.

- Purchase a bulletin board and attach recent pictures of the family.

- Frame and hang a picture of the care recipient over his/her bed. A picture taken when he/she was young and vibrant. (It made my Mom so proud each time someone said how beautiful she was.)

- Check and see that he/she has an adequate supply of allowed snacks.

- Purchase a radio and put it on a station he/she likes to listen to. (Then, only the "ON"/"OFF" knob had to be turned to "ON.")

- Purchase a beautiful notebook for visitors to sign. (This even helps the caregiver to check on who has been in for a visit.)

- Foster closeness by giving your loved one a weekly manicure. It provides "private time" to talk and to make personal contact with one another.

- If your care recipient is living at home alone, make certain all medicines can easily be opened. Write out IN BIG LETTERS the quantities and times each medication must be taken.

- Help remove facial hair — this is a constant worry.

- Make certain hair is always washed and well groomed.

- Do not visit at the same time if your loved one is in a nursing home. Check in at different and varied times to make certain your loved one is getting proper care all day long — not just during anticipated visits.

CONCLUSION

To the Reader:

Always remember this quotation:

The opposite of Love is not Hate — but Indifference.

People filling out this book to help make their loved ones' lives a little easier are certainly not "Indifferent."

God Bless and Good Luck!

Trust me, filling out this book, and giving it to your future "caregivers" is the best gift in the whole world. We all need "peace of mind."

Dee Marrella

Dee Marrella
Contact Information
610-288-5801 (fax)
info@focusonethics.com(e-mail)
www.focusonethics.com

RED ALERT

Note: Take a half dozen sheets of 8 1/2" x 11" blank paper and recreate the RED ALERT list found on the next two pages. Fill in one of the sheets completely, fold it and place it in the rear of this guide book so that the top of the sheet and the words RED ALERT can be easily seen. The words RED ALERT should be visible above the pages of the book and to anyone who finds this book. The information on this RED ALERT is critical information that you would want anyone who found you to have quick access.

On this page I am listing **Very Important** information about myself. Please refer to it when any emergency   situation arises.

My Social Security #: _____

My Birth date and current age: _____

I am allergic to the following drugs:

_____

_____

_____

I am allergic to the following foods:

_____

_____

I AM being treated for (fill in with illness, condition, disease, i.e, Diabetes): _____

_____

_____

_____

My Personal Physician is:

Name: _____

Address: _____

Telephone #: _____

My Pharmacy is:

Name: _____

Address: _____

Telephone #: _____

NOTE: Create these RED ALERT forms and have them ready for use at any time. Keep the most current version of this form folded with the "RED ALERT" facing out and inserted into the back of this guide.

PART X
Notes

NOTES

LIFE'S LESSONS

NOTES

NOTES

LIFE'S LESSONS

NOTES

NOTES

NOTES

NOTES

LIFE'S LESSONS

NOTES

NOTES

NOTES

NOTES

NOTES

NOTES

NOTES

NOTES

NOTES

NOTES